YOGA JOURNEY

A Personal Experience

Walter Lovelace

authorHOUSE®

AuthorHouse™ UK
1663 Liberty Drive
Bloomington, IN 47403   USA
www.authorhouse.co.uk
Phone: 0800.197.4150

Published by AuthorHouse 09/27/2016

ISBN: 978-1-5246-6397-1 (sc)
ISBN: 978-1-5246-6396-4 (e)

All is Energy

Albert Einstein

Yoga is Science of the Mind

Sri Patanjali

ACKNOWLEDGEMENTS AND PREFACE

My interest in Indian philosophy, yoga sessions and meditation have all been encouraged by studying, discussing and recording a large number of experiences with many fellow yoga enthusiasts in Stockholm. Many leaders have the remarkable ability to infuse every yoga session with an awareness of body, mind and spirit in unison. Their sessions are not just a number of postures but a unique confirmation that the ancient Indian philosophy of yoga still offers a path to inner consciousness. But I probably wouldn't have written this book if I hadn't met up with Ratheesh Mani. He encouraged me to dive into Indian philosophy and the Indian way of thinking. Namaste Ratheesh!

I must thank my daughter Heléne for her sharp comments after reading the draft and also for her lovely photographs.

I have of course gleaned many sources of information from books and WEB sites and none of the authors is responsible for any mistakes I may have made or my interpretation of their works. My list of Reference Literature has been the main source of inspiration.

● ●

Some yoga workshops in Stockholm and retreats in India confirmed my ambition to try and investigate what is so attractive to millions of yoga students all over the world. Yoga is now rapidly being introduced to school children. Sessions are also held in prisons and hospitals and there is now a style available to every kind of society, even Green Yoga. Virtually every TV talk show has interviewed yoga teachers and one can maybe ask what more is there to talk about. Yoga has become big business. However, behind the scene of apparent satisfaction with modern yoga there is now a growing awareness that the original ideas from India like Ahimsa and Aparigraha (Non-violence and not stealing or accumulation of excess wealth) are once again becoming relevant to our way of living. The study of an inner consciousness has been a central theme of Indian yoga philosophy for centuries. The Mahatma Gandhi, Nelson Mandela and Martin Luther King were all involved in a vigorous and active search for oneness in humanity. So perhaps the search for consciousness or oneness can also be part of the everyday yoga experience.

I have tried to re-trace my own experiences during my yoga journey. My confrontation with yoga history, philosophy, mantras and meditation has contributed to my appreciation of what consciousness means. For several years I was an active member of the Humanist Stockholm organization where I first became aware that religion can stand in the way of spirituality. Also that a personal spirituality based on yoga philosophy can allow one to dive much deeper into a present awareness than organized religion.

During the latter half of 2015 I became extremely ill and could not practice yoga postures at all. Meditation kept me going but I had extreme pain and fatigue for six months. Slowly I have had to start practicing asanas from the beginning again. Yoga has been a great help and confirmed once again that yoga is not just for the very young and healthy but rather a way of living for anyone at any time.

INTRODUCTION

This is not a book about how to practise yoga postures but rather an approach as to how to include a search for consciousness in every aspect of yoga. Our yoga journey is the tool for understanding.

My yoga journey started more than ten years ago with an intense and dedicated interest in learning yoga postures from Ashtanga, Hatha, Jivamukti, etc. In the beginning I practised most days of the week and imagined that I would never tire, in spite of long trips to the studio in the early hours of the morning. A pleasant reward was that my blood pressure dropped back to normal and I could stop taking medicines. So, from the start, I knew that yoga could provide health benefits as well as an enormous feeling of wellbeing. No matter how tired and fed-up one felt at the beginning of a session, the mental lift afterwards was deeply satisfying. Meditation, Savasana, or corpse posture, wound up every session so it also became clear that postures or asanas were only part of the remedy. Meditation and yoga practise from the very beginning fired my interest in searching for an inner consciousness. This is an easily misunderstood word and means many different things to many different people. Some will associate it with awareness, or mindfulness or how part of the mind works. I am interested in tracing the experience of consciousness back to the origins of yoga. Equally important, I want to know how consciousness affects our everyday practise of yoga.

The nature of consciousness was investigated in the ancient Indian text called the Upanisad where our life experience was thought to have four states of mind: The Self Awake, The Self Dreaming, The Self in Dreamless Sleep and The Super Conscious Self. In the early days when Indian philosophy was first introduced to our western way of thought many famous people were attracted to these ideas. For example, Somerset Maugham, Christopher Isherwood, Aldous Huxley, Dr Albert Schweitzer and many more. The famous Sanskrit expression from the Upanisad "Tat twam asi" meaning That Thou Art Thyself (That man must see himself in all beings and see all beings in himself) has provided an introduction for many people to the study of yoga and consciousness.

Nowadays, the study of neuroscience has made enormous advances into the true nature of the brain and how the mind works. However, most studies are based on the operating functions of the brain and no one has yet unearthed exactly what consciousness is and where it exists. If one is a religious person then the dualistic idea of body and soul still prevails. Alternatively, the concept of body and mind may be more attractive. If consciousness is the result of continuous brain activity and disappears on death then there is still the option of refining and enjoying the experience while living.

The fascinating book Biocentrism by Robert Lanza and Bob Berman suggests that life and consciousness are the keys to understanding the true nature of the universe; that life and consciousness creates the universe and not the other way around. This concept has been applauded and debunked by equally famous scientists but Biocentrism has obvious similarities to some of the ideas in Indian philosophy.

Practising yoga postures alone was not enough for me, so over the past two years I have started to record my experiences of yoga sessions, meditation and my study of Indian philosophy. Many yoga students loose interest when coming face to face with the enormous diversity of knowledge from India. Blind religious faith is confused with philosophy and is not attractive to our secular societies. Mythology, religion and philosophy have a very complex history in India and it is easy to confuse one with the other. New Age ideas make matters worse and it is easy to give up the quest for understanding. On the other hand Quantum Physics and modern neuroscience has opened the door to a new approach in trying to experience and understand consciousness.

Presumably most yoga students sense at times that there is an inner meaning to be found when practising postures or meditation. If my own Yoga Journey helps others to sort things out and lead on to deeper studies then it has been worthwhile. The journey is always everything.

Walter Lovelace, Stockholm September 2016

CHAPTER ONE

Yoga History and Traditions

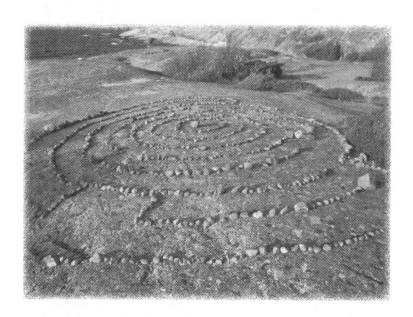

The single most important aspect of YOGA is that our physical asana practise is just one part of YOGA SCIENCE. The Yoga Sutras of Patanjali make this perfectly clear when defining yoga as Science of

1

the Mind. This mental science is founded on Raja Yoga. The Sutras provide a firm foundation for all of the many types of yoga postures and meditation which have been developed over the centuries. They all have one thing in common, the search for and development of a particular state of being we call consciousness. The asanas, or postures together with pranayama, which is the meditative technique of breath awareness, help us to prepare the body for the more difficult work in opening up the subliminal or unconsciousness mind.

The subject of yoga history is enormous, difficult to define and open to a number of interpretations. However, we can make it easier by noting that the main elements of philosophy in India are The Vedas, Brahmanism, Hinduism, Jainism, Buddhism and Sikhism. Yoga history has evolved over thousands of years and can be very roughly covered and studied over four periods: Vedic, Pre-Classical, Classical and Post-Classical.

Brahmanism and modern day Hinduism were founded on the Vedas which are probably the oldest Yogic texts known to man. The Upanisads and the Bhagavad-Gita texts belong to the Pre-Classical times. The Patanjali Yoga Sutras were assembled during the Classical period and are the first attempt to summarise Classical Yoga with about 200 aphorisms or sutras. These "Threads" refer to the principles of Raja Yoga. It is here that we find the eightfold limbs of yoga or Ashtanga. The Hatha Pradipika was introduced in the 15th century or Post Classical period. Present day yoga has little to do with trying to escape reality but rather concentrates on accepting oneself and focussing on living with the moment. It is usually recognised that yoga came to the Western World in 1893 at the World Parliament of Religions in Chicago. Since then yoga has slowly evolved into something that provides alternative solutions to vast numbers of people. Yoga seems to answer a need from both sick and healthy.

Today, we have many yoga styles from all over the world. Each one provides an alternative series of asanas, mantras, meditation, etc. They have been introduced to suit a particular need or fashion or age group. Yoga is also used for medicinal purposes, such as aches and pains, headaches, anxiety, stress, high blood pressure etc. Together with Ayurveda food recipes, yoga can present a number of solutions to better health. The vast body of literature on yoga makes it perfectly clear that interpretations and practises have varied from school to school and teacher to teacher over many years. For most of us, however, when we practise yoga we have chosen a series of asanas which we find worthwhile and attractive. The student may want to experiment with other styles as time and opportunity allows. One should remember that there is no single correct form of yoga. We all have our favourite style which happens to be the yogic path that suits us at the time.

Historically, we can see that it is only in recent times that there has been an intensive concentration on the physical practise.

The following list of yoga styles is just one effort to describe what is generally available in Europe, USA and other countries. There are many variations of these styles, especially today in the USA, but most of them follow the principles laid down at an early age.

- **HATHA** as practised today is the oldest of styles which include physical asanas. Literally, the union of the sun and moon or opposites.
- **ASHTANGA** is demanding and includes a specific flow of different postures. Literally, the eight limbed yoga.
- **VINYASA** has specific movements with controlled and linked breathing.
  Literally, breathing and movement.
- **YIN** ensures that energy, stamina and awareness come to a balance in the body. Literally, the passive concept of yin.
- **KUNDALINI** includes asanas, meditation, mantras and breath control.
  Literally, a coiled snake.
- **JIVAMUKTI** is a stimulating style based on Hatha with powerful asanas and music. Literally, the awakened individual.
- **IYENGAR** is a highly disciplined practise that creates a balance in the body. Literally, yoga developed by BKS Iyengar.
- **ANUSARA** combines Tantra with calming asanas.
  Literally, following your heart.

These yoga styles focus mainly on the body and asanas; nonetheless they all offer the opportunity of experiencing something more than just physical exercise. They all affect our psyche and work on our consciousness. Working with concentration on a particular posture requires that all other thoughts are excluded so that mind and body become one.

There are six limbs of yoga that pay more attention to the transcendental nature of the mind; Raja Yoga, Hatha Yoga, Bhakthi Yoga, Jnana Yoga Mantra Yoga and Karma Yoga. They all lead to a greater understanding of and search for wisdom.

An interesting form of contemporary yoga which deserves further study is Green Yoga. Georg and Brenda Feuerstein have explained in their book "Green Yoga" that this concept continues the ancient ideals and essence of Hinduism found in the Bhagavad-Gita. In practise this demands that the core values of yoga are applied to preservation of the natural environment.

The Upanisads have been a source of inspiration and solace for generations. They followed on from the Vedas and are sometimes called the Vedanta – meaning the end of the Vedas. One can say that they are dedicated to the inner life with advice on leadership, solace, enjoyment and wisdom. Most important, they seek to find answers to the eternal questions; "Who am I?" "What am I?" "What makes me?" and, not least, "What makes my ears to hear, my eyes to see and my mind to think?" These questions which are now the subject of serious neurological scientists fascinated many famous people in the 1920s when Hindu philosophy came in contact with western ideas. The interest was so great in the USA that the Vedanta Society was started in Southern California. For the student there are many books and commentaries available.

Perhaps we can summarize the history and tradition of yoga as a centuries-long growing awareness that the highest reality is only to be found in an inner consciousness. Therefore it is only natural that we apply yoga asanas, pranayama and meditation in order to heighten this consciousness. This does not lead to isolation from the outside world but rather to the realisation that we can live a more worthy life when practising yoga. If we are observant, we can carry this way of thinking into every aspect of our lives. Hopefully, this quieter and more sympathetic attitude towards others will result in a better world. Yoga of today can lead on to a search for oneness in humanity.

CHAPTER TWO

Mythology Religion Philosophy

According to the Supreme Court of India the Hindu religion does not claim any one prophet, does not worship any one god, does not believe in any one philosophical concept, does not follow any one act of religious rite and does not satisfy the traditional features of a religion or creed. It is a way of life and nothing more. India is a secular state and does not have a state religion.

The distinction between philosophy and religion is not clear in Hinduism and the Sanskrit language does not have exact equivalents for these European terms.

Evidence of mythology can be seen and experienced all over India. The Hindu gods and goddesses are everywhere, in wayside carvings, shrines and temples, etc. But they are also depicted in posters and advertisements, amulets, jewellery and in TV shows. For somebody from the West it is a surprise, almost a shock, when entering a temple for the first time to see paper posters on the walls illustrating the gods alongside exquisite stone carvings. Supposedly these paper prints are only meant to be reminders of the divine. They are so deeply woven into the fabric of life that Hinduism is impossible to imagine without them.

It is impossible to study or travel in India without becoming aware of the constant presence of mythology. Countless Indian myths, fables or stories have had a profound impact on everyday life. Myths are morality tales and have always been a way of trying to explain unusual happenings, pain, death, the miracle of birth, ethics and morals etc. The Indian myths are always present; unlike the Christian myths which are assumed by many to be historical events.

Indian myths can be of help in understanding the history of yoga and where the strange names of postures have originated. They also abound in the countless mantras. At the very least they provide fascinating and entertaining stories about the birth of Indian religion and philosophy.

One fascinating aspect of myths and religion in India is that they are not without criticism by well-known Indian thinkers and have been adapted to Western thought and philosophy. For example, the famous Hindu Brahmin, Ram Mohan Roy, who in 1828 formed the Brahmo Samaj in order to promote ethical monotheism and which he maintained was rooted in the Upanisads. He prohibited images of gods and goddesses in Samaj buildings and initiated many reforms for the benefit of both women and men.

Anyway, on a lighter note, one can see that modern men and women in India say that cricket is the new religion and that famous cricketers like Sachin Tendulkar are the new gods!

Yoga is just one of the six classical schools of Indian Philosophy. When practising yoga asanas it is helpful to try and understand a little about the spiritual background of these traditions. It will then become clear for a sincere seeker that there is a difference between the authentic Indian teachings and the modern teaching of postures.

- **Yoga** (Practical Methods to deepen the experience of consciousness)
- **Samkhya** (Self-realization through knowing the difference between spirit and matter)
- **Vedanta** (Contemplative Self-Inquiry)
- **Vaisheshika** (Physical Sciences)
- **Nyaya** (A system of Logic or Reasoning)
- **Mimasa** (Freedom Through Action)

More detail can be found in the REFERENCE SOURCES at the end of this book. However, something should be said here about the Upanisads. The word Upanisad can be translated from Sanskrit to mean "To sit down near the guru." From sad(to sit), upa(near to), and ni(down). They represent a break with the materialistic view of life to a belief that there is a spiritual core common to everything.

There seems to be a continuous process in India of weaving all of the elements of various religious philosophies, mythology and religions into a fabric of common acceptance by the people. Religious philosophy is more like a way of life in India than in other countries and more aligned to family traditions than to the state. India has retained its unique ancient traditions, customs and festivals which are all deeply entrenched in history.

Our yoga practise is rooted in yoga philosophy and no matter which style we choose it is almost impossible to escape from the idea that there is a deeper meaning in it than just physical exercise. However, it should be remembered that any attempt to analyse the question about religion or philosophy is influenced by our religious spectacles. If we have a Christian upbringing then we will tend to judge Indian ways by Christian thinking and history. Even if we are atheists or agnostics we still belong to societies that are grounded in a thousand years of Christian religion. We have to take a step from the outside and although extremely difficult we have to make an attempt to understand the inside perspective held by Indian people.

Yoga philosophy, like all other philosophies, has to be considered whether it supports life affirmation or life negation. It seems to me that in India both forms have been supported for countless years but that very few of us in the West are aware that there is a choice which can lead on to a commitment. I suppose that I could, like many others who practise yoga regularly, just enjoy the postures and meditation and not bother about consciousness. However, it is always tempting to go a step further and to explore the very boundaries of our birth, life and death. Anyhow, if nothing else, the search can make everyday life more meaningful.

CHAPTER THREE

We Need Some Sanskrit

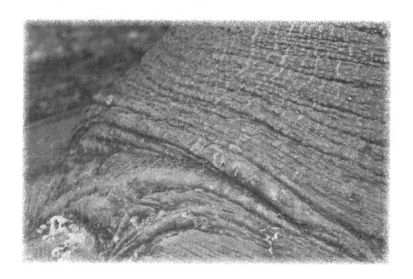

The language of Yoga is Sanskrit. This ancient language is now drawing attention from universities and scholars all over the world and also from the thousands of men and women practicing yoga. Children and teenagers are at an early age also coming in contact with Sanskrit through yoga classes.

Hindi is the most widely spoken language but India has a population of more than one billion people and has 18 official languages and numerous lesser ones. Both Hindi and Sanskrit are written in the Devanagari alphabet. English has incorporated many words from all of these languages like Brahmin, Mantra, Karma, Cot, Loot, Thug, Chintz, Bandanna, Dungaree, Rajah, Pundit, Coolie, Chutney, Juggernaut, Mulligatawny, Teak, Copra, Atoll, Tourmaline, Beriberi, Serendipity, Bungalow, Cushy, Guru, Bangle, Punch, Shampoo, Chit, Calico, Char etc.

Sanskrit, meaning refined or perfected, is the classical language of ancient India and dates back thousands of years. It is very important in India because the ancient Vedas and other Hindu texts are in this language.

We know that Sanskrit, yoga and mantra have been an integral part of Indian life for many years and include a multitude of traditions, practices, approaches and cultures. Yoga came to the Western World in 1893 and since then there has evolved many, many, different styles. However, they all have one thing in common; they are all concerned with consciousness. Fortunately, the novice does not have to rigorously study Sanskrit or the entire history of yoga, we just have to do it and enjoy. There are some excellent Sanskrit resources on the WEB. The following Sanskrit words are useful to memorize since they are frequently in use.

Suryanamaskar	Sun Salutation
Samasthiti	Standing Evenly
Tadasana	Mountain Posture
Uttanasana	Forward Bend
Ardha Mandalasana	Lunge
Adho Mukha Svanasana	Downward Facing Dog
Chaturanga Dandasana	Four Limb Staff
Urdhva Mukha Svanasana	Upward Facing Dog
Savasana	Corpse Posture
Yama	Moral Discipline
Niyama	Self-Restraint
Asana	Posture
Pranayama	Breath Control
Pratyahara	Sense-Withdrawal
Dharana	Concentration
Dhyana	Meditation
Samadhi	Ecstasy
Satya	Truth
Satyagraha	Commitment to the truth
Ahimsa	Non-violence and respect for life
Surya	The sun
Namaskara	Greetings
Namaste	Hello, I greet you
Karma Yoga	Discipline of action
Kama	Desire and passion
Atman	Inner-self and consciousness
Hari Om	Salutations (Or perhaps, Hari is Om)
Brahman	Absolute Reality
Brahmin	Ritual Specialist
Brahmana	Vedic Texts
Brahma	Hindu Deity

direct contact with the inner self. Ashtanga Yoga is derived from the Patanjali system called Raja Yoga.

Having studied some yoga history, the principles of Hatha, Ashtanga and Iyengar, I started thinking about how to approach the sequencing of postures. Since posture is important I decided to try and aim for feelings of well-being, joy and balance in everything.

In the beginning, my movements and postures tended to be hasty and uncoordinated. After successive cycles I found that I could gradually reduce the time and energy spent on each position. My breath started to align with the shape of movements and I started to experience a continuous flow between each one. True sequencing had started.

I soon realised that in order to try and understand a cycle of, for example, Sun Salutation, I needed knowledge and experience of Pranayama, Meditation and Yoga Philosophy. They all contributed to establishing a slow, rhythmic flowing motion that brought me closer to my inner self.

My final aim was to try and understand the following:

What is true knowledge or wisdom?
What is true freedom?
What is true happiness?

This enlightenment can only be achieved by the inner self. I was now becoming more aware of the Eight

Limbs of Yoga. The first two can be summarised as follows:

YAMAS

- **Ahimsa** Non-violence and respect for life
- **Satya** Commitment to the truth
- **Asteya** Non-stealing
- **Brahmacharya** Merging with spiritual oneness
- **Aparigraha** Abstention from greed

NYAMAS

- **Shaucha** Purity
- **Santosha** Contentment
- **Tapas** Burning Enthusiasm and self-discipline
- **Swadhyaya** Self-study
- **Ishvaraapranidhana** Dedication to the Absolute

Perhaps the most difficult precept to practise is Ahimsa to oneself. This is where our yoga practise can be a great help by not judging ourselves too harshly.

Surya Namaskara

The Surya Namaskara or Sun Salutation is traditionally practised in India in the early morning, facing the sun. Mind, body and spirit are combined into a harmonious exercise for the enjoyment of everyone. Asanas and pranayama are united in the process. Ordinary breathing can be replaced by Conscious Breathing.

There are twelve spinal positions where the spine and ligaments are stretched backwards and forwards. Blood circulation is improved and toxins are removed by the blood and sweat. This invigorating exercise removes stiffness and dryness in the limbs. Movements must be slow and graceful without jerking at any time.

Practising the Sun Salutation together with the Gayatri Mantra can be an incredible experience. They support each other and fuse together. I soon realised that I could combine the ancient and lengthy twelve Surya Namaskara mantra names with the twelve postures. The combined effect is very slow and very graceful since each posture has to be held for the length of each phrase. For example,"Om Hraam Mitraya Namaha." This lengthy mantra with the Sun Salutation postures soon became my favourite and was sufficient for a complete morning session.

Conscious Breathing

Initially, Conscious Breathing was necessary to enable the sears in India to chant in rhythm. Chanting and repeating the Vedic hymns was the only way people could remember the words. The Rishis or sears collected a vast amount of information and made up a system and catalogued it into a number of books, now called the Vedas. At that time, the country of India incorporated parts of Tibet, Mongolia and Afghanistan. The Vedas include, therefore, considerable influence from other countries. The people of India have years of experience and Pranayama has been more important than the asanas. The physical practise of asanas is still relatively unknown. On the other hand, Yoga Philosophy is integrated with the way of life in India.

Chakras

One way in establishing a slow rhythmic movement is to concentrate on the chakras. I started by learning the main five focus points where energy is collected in the body. These are called Chakras. Gliding slowly through each point and hesitating momentarily it is much easier to reach a pleasant routine.

1. Behind the Pubic Bone
2. Behind the Navel
3. Behind the Solar Plexus
4. Behind the Chest
5. Behind the Throat

Conscious Breathing can be learnt by counting, 1-2-3-4-5, or by naming the Chakras. It is important to start the inhaling and exhaling at the pubic bone and always finishing with the throat. We can practise it by reciting out loud and by visualising the Chakras. Holding the breath is beneficial so one can extend the practise by lengthening the pause after the count of five.

CHAPTER FIVE

Mantras are of Help

Mantra chanting has a long history in India. Perhaps the most famous mantra is the enigmatic "OM". Like a poem, a mantra can express ideas which go far beyond the very words. Chanting a mantra together with others provides a group identity and encourages a meditative attitude. A mantra is sometimes called yoga for the mind

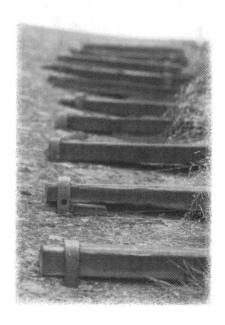

and affects consciousness by the words, the rhythm and whether it is repeated loudly, softly or silently. Mantras can also be seen as a media for meditation.

There are Indian mantras for every occasion in our daily lives, sunrise, sunset, before eating, peaceful sleeping, practising yoga asanas etc.

GAYATRI MANTRA

Om bhur bhuvah svah
Tat savitur varenyam
Bhargo devasya dhimahi
Dhiyo yo nah prachodayat

"Let us meditate on the light of the sun which represents spiritual consciousness and may our thoughts be inspired by that divine light".

There are several gayatri mantras but this one is the oldest and most well-known. There is a famous metaphor in Hinduism which explains a great deal about how they see the universe: "The sun equals light which equals knowledge which equals consciousness."

SHANTI MANTRA

Om saha navavatu
Saha nau bhunaktu
Saha viryam karavaavahai
Tejasvi naavadhitamastu maa vidvishaavahai
OM shanti, shanti, shanti

"Together may we be protected and nourished and work with great energy. Let our journey together be brilliant and effective. May there be no bad feelings between us. Peace, peace, peace."

GURU MANTRA

Gurur Brahma Gurur Vishnu
Gurur devo Maheshwarah
Gurur saakshaat para brahma
Tasmai Shri Gurave namaha

"Guru is Brahma. Guru is Vishnu. Guru is Maheshwara (Shiva). Guru is Supreme Brahman Itself. Respect unto that Guru". This can be interpreted that it is the knowledge itself that comes from Brahma, Vishnu etc. which is Guru.

MAHAMRITYUNJAYA MANTRA

OM tryambakam yajamahe
Sugandhim pusti-vardhanam
Urvarukamiva bandhanan
Mrtyormuksiya mamrtat

"We meditate on the three-eyed reality of creation, existence and dissolution."
(Note – short version)

SLEEP MANTRA

Om Agasti Shayinah. Om Agasti Shayinah. Om Agasti Shayinah. Om Agasti Shayinah.

Agastya was a famous sage and healer from ancient India and this mantra is the perfect lullaby when sung slower and slower and quieter and quieter. After five minutes even the most restless child or stressed person will find profound and deep relaxation and sleep.

HARI OM or OM OM OM OM

Yoga Asana students chant the mantra OM or AUM with every session, usually at the beginning and end. OM has been handed down by the sages of India since many thousands of years ago. It is said to represent Primordial Vibration and can be found in all living and material things. It is used in all religions and by all civilisations. OM is mentioned in the Upanisads, in the Bhagavad Gita and in many other texts from India.

Modern science says that every atom and every molecule is formed by energy vibration. OM is perhaps found in everything in the universe.

Most of us get acquainted with mantras during some of our yoga courses. However, there are many opportunities to deepen the knowledge by attending special mantra lessons as well as gatherings dedicated to chanting. Mantras can be spoken, chanted or silently repeated. It is not advisable just to repeat the words as a rigid discipline. It soon becomes boring. A counting scheme with or without mala beads can provide the necessary introduction to a pleasant routine. After a while one will become aware that a mantra can open the way towards more profound relaxation and meditation. This is perhaps the main reason for getting involved with mantras.

SUN SALUTATION

We have all practised a Sun Salutation and maybe some of us have tried out the repetition of 108 continuous sun salutations. There is however a special charm in combining it with a mantra. The Gayatri Mantra is an obvious first choice. The following combination is very slow and graceful and gives plenty of time to complete each movement. There are 12 mantras and each posture is held for the entire length of each salutation phrase. No short cuts! I usually practise six rounds very slowly.

Surya Namaskara (Sun Salutation mantra for Asana Practise)

1	Om Hraam Mitraya Namah	EXHALE	Prayer Posture
2	Om Hreem Ravaye Namah	INHALE	Raised Arms
3	Om Hroom Suryaya Namah	EXHALE	Hands to Feet
4	Om Hraim Bhanave Namah	INHALE	Bent knee Lunge
5	Om Hraum Khagaya Namah	HOLD	Plank Posture
6	Om Hrah Pushne Namah	EXHALE	Knees, chest, chin to floor
7	Om Hraam Hiranyagarbha Namah	INHALE	Cobra Posture
8	Om Hreem Marichaye Namah	EXHALE	Downward Facing Dog
9	Om Hroom Adityaya Namah	INHALE	Bent knee Lunge
10	Om Hraim Savitre Namah	EXHALE	Hands to Feet
11	Om Hraum Arkaya Namah	INHALE	Raised Arms
12	Om Hrah Bhaskaraya Namah	EXHALE	Prayer Posture

Surya, or the sun, has twelve names (Mitraya, Ravaye, Suryaya, Bhanave, Khagaya, Pushne, Hiranyagarbhaya, Marichaye, Adityaya, Savitre, Arkaya, Bhaskaraya). They are associated with the six repeated mantras (Hraam, Hreem, Hroom, Hraim, Hraum, Hrah). Namah stands for Salutation. The meaning of each Salute is related to different aspects of the sun, shining, creation, nourishment etc.

Of course a pleasant alternative, especially at home, is to practise the postures to chant music. One can then concentrate on the postures alone. There are several CDs available.

CHAPTER SIX

Pranayama is Life Bringing

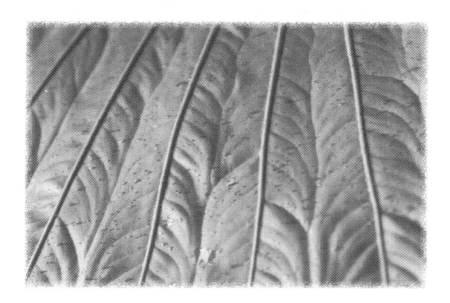

Pranayama is the fourth stage of yoga according to Patanjali and regulates breath, energy and oxygen uptake. The meditative purpose of breath awareness helps to clear the mind of clutter. I made it a routine with home practise to try and start every yoga session with at least one of the following sessions.

BENDING AND BREATHING

Take up a kneeling position and sit between, or on, the heels

- Left hand on right wrist behind back- Breathe in
- Breathe out and lower head to floor. Count to ten
- Rise and breathe in
- Repeat ten times
- Right hand to left wrist and repeat the sequence but start with an out-breath

NADI SHODHANA (Alternate Nostril Breathing)

Sit in lotus or a comfortable position. Place right-hand thumb and ring finger on nostrils

- Close right nostril with thumb and count 4
- Breathe in and count 4 with left nostril
- Close both nostrils for 2
- Close left and breathe out for 4 with right. Close both nostrils for 2
- Breathe in through right nostril for count 4
- Close both nostrils for count 2
- Close right and breathe out of left nostril for count 4

Repeat the entire sequence three times.

KAPALABHATI (Breath of Fire)

Spread out legs with soft knees and feet at 45 degrees

- Squat low down, back straight
- Draw stomach in sharply, blowing out through nose, first slowly then rapidly for 30 times
- Take a few deep breaths and on the last exhale retain the breath for as long as possible

After having taken a few normal breaths repeat the entire sequence three times.

There are at least 100 classical breathing techniques. For example, Ujjayi (The Psychic Breath), Brahmari, (The Bees Breath) and Sitali (Tongue Hissing). Many forms of meditation are based on the foundation of breath awareness. However, it is easier to establish one routine that can be enjoyed regularly rather than trying to remember several.

There is a long history of breathing practises from India and the routines have therefore been adapted to suit diverse occasions. For example **KAPALABHATI** can be carried out sitting in a chair or sitting cross legged on the studio floor. Neither one is necessarily the only correct routine. The occasion must be allowed to determine the desirable routine. It is important that the environment is calm and relaxed.

CHAPTER SEVEN

Meditation is the Reward

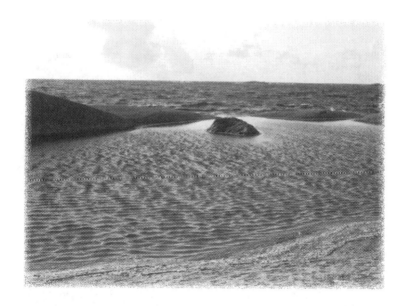

C orpse pose, or Savasana, is a restorative posture that is difficult to master. The main idea behind this posture is to practise letting go of all the distractions cluttering the mind in such a way that we can begin to experience a kind of conscious dying. The lengthy process involved can take months or years to achieve but leads the way towards rewarding meditation.

Total relaxation under conscious control of the mind has to start at the very beginning of lying down on the yoga mat. In fact, lying down and getting up with ease and gracefulness is part of the initial process. It is worth practising these movements so that rolling onto the mat and rolling up can be carried out smoothly and seamlessly.

After several years of practise I found myself automatically checking out how I should tune into Savasana. When practising at home it's a good idea to establish a solid routine. The following is useful when getting started.

- Dimmed lighting
- Relaxing music can be helpful
- Supports under the head and knees and feet wide apart
- A covering blanket
- Eye bags or scarf if needed
- Hands facing palm upwards
- Letting mother earth embrace the entire body
- Yielding to earth with head, shoulders, limbs etc.
- Letting the skin around the eyes, lips and forehead be softened
- Awareness on all body parts, no need to concentrate

- Normal breathing
- Letting go for at least ten minutes

Meditation

Most of the time we are at the mercy of our senses and everyone who has tried to meditate experiences this immediately. Every sound, every thought and every movement interferes with our concentration no matter how hard we try to resist. This is quite normal because the brain has evolved this way and is continually checking for differences that are presented by the five senses. We seem to be forced to have to follow every impulse that enters our awareness. After long practise we can try to disregard at least some of these distractions. Meditation is the practise of inhibiting the senses, as best we can. There are many ways we can try and assist in this process. For example, breath control and sitting tall and straight in lotus posture help a great deal.

It may take a lifetime to achieve but the ultimate goal is not only letting go of distracting thoughts but also becoming acutely aware and sharp in mind at the same time. There is a famous saying from the KATHA UPANISAD which has been translated into English as; "The sharp edge of a razor is difficult to pass over." In other words, the process of meditation and finding Samadhi is very difficult. Fortunately, most of us begin to experience a calmer mind from the very beginning since we are usually stressed out with daily problems and experiences. Even a short period of daily meditation will bring a wonderful feeling of well-being.

It is important to remember that true meditation cannot be entered into by reading instructions. Meditation has to be experienced and this takes time to achieve. It is only by, repeatedly, throwing out every disturbance caused by the five senses that we can come close to entering that state of mind which opens up the way to glorious nothingness. Every time we fail just means that we have been given the opportunity to start again on a new inward voyage. With every new attempt, we can take a step forward. (More brain cells!)

The following advice may help us to get started but each and every one of us will surely discover his or her way to "pass over the razors edge" and find true peace of mind. First, after having experienced it just a little will we know "That it was that." The famous expression "The Veil Was Lifted" is another way of looking at this state of awareness.

- Asanas and pranayama are helpful in preparing the mind for meditation
- Meditation can be practised in a seated position, or lying down
- The seated position must be firm and stable. A bolster or blanket helps
- It is advisable to spend some time in finding the calmest way of sitting

- If you have to adjust the body come immediately back to the focused breath
- It is natural to drift away, but you can always return to the breath
- Always, follow the breath
- Try to meditate at least for ten minutes
- Try not to judge your own criticism, just return to the breath
- Allow time to return slowly, using the five senses once again
- Carry the new calmness with you throughout the day
- Let no one or nothing disturb your inner peace

True meditation cannot be properly learnt from a book. Unfortunately, circumstances may make it impossible for some of us to find a guru, leader or teacher. However, nothing can stop us from attempting to follow meditation at home or in a hospital bed. Having learnt the possibilities that are offered with meditation will encourage the search for a deeper understanding.

Yoga Nidra Meditation

Some time ago I discovered Yoga Nidra or psychic relaxation. The body is fully awake when the mind goes into deep conscious sleep.

There are many CD:s and courses available and perhaps it is advisable to find a qualified teacher before trying out Yoga Nidra.

The following list provides an introduction into what to expect when practising Yoga Nidra. There are many different methods, so the list just highlights one such approach.

Yoga Nidra

- **Lie in Savasana**, pause. Close eyes, pause. Be aware and listen, pause. I will not sleep, pause. Deep breathing, pause. Breathing out, say Relax. Be aware of distant sounds. Scan for more sounds, pause. Even indoor sounds, pause. Be aware and visualise the room, pause. Total awareness of body on floor, pause. Feel how body interfaces with floor, pause. No concentration. Listen and be aware of the breath. Mentally say: I am going to practise Yoga Nidra.
- Make a Sankalpa (Resolution)
- **Rotation of consciousness**. Very quickly jump from point to point. Be aware.

- Start with right hand. Fingers, wrist, elbow, shoulder, armpit, waist, hip, thigh, knee, calf, ankle, heel, sole, toes,
- Left hand etc
- Back. Right shoulder, left, shoulder blades, buttocks, spine, back.
- Front. Top of head, forehead, eyebrows, eyes, ears, cheeks, nose, lips, chin, throat, collarbone, chests, navel, abdomen
- Major parts. Whole of legs, arms, back, front, head, Whole Body. Long pause.
- **Breathing**. Be aware of in and out breathing, pause. Feel breath from navel to throat. UP on Inhalation, DOWN on exhalation, pause. Feel body expand on IN and relax on OUT. Repeat and then long pause.
- **Visualization**. I AM AWAKE. Be aware of manipura chakra in solar plexus behind the navel. On exhale feel energy gathering in manipura, pause. Inhale and feel energy streaming to all body parts. Repeat and long pause.
- **Symbols**. Awareness to the space in front of eyes, pause. Blue skies, golden sun, fountains, lotus flowers, stars. Dive into the sea; find a green jewel which explodes into light.
- **Focus on space in front of eyes.** Watch the darkness without involvement.
- Pause and let go with complete awareness. Long pause.

- **Sankalpa.** Repeat and pause.
- **Finish**. Become aware of breathing, pause. Relaxation, pause. Be aware of the room and body parts. Stretch arms and legs. Open eyes and rest in Lotus position. Carry the experience with you for the rest of the day.

In his book *A Map of Mental States* John H. Clark characterized meditation or Dhyana as a method by which a person concentrates more and more upon less and less. The aim is to empty the mind while, paradoxically, remaining alert. It sounds easy but takes most of us several years to accomplish.

CHAPTER EIGHT

Ancient Indian Literature

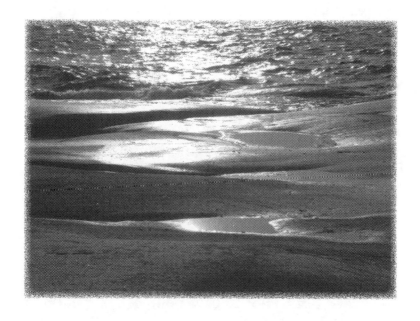

The enormous volume of ancient literature from India, often written as aphorisms in sutras, makes it difficult to know where to start and how to decide what to select. I thought that the Patanjali texts were probably the easiest to understand and therefor concentrated on the translation and commentary by Sri Swami Satchidananda.

None the less, it is fascinating and rewarding to try and capture an overall picture of the principal Hindu texts. After all, they are the very foundation on which yoga is built.

The Vedas

There are four main collections of Veda texts known as the Rigveda, the Samaveda, the Yajurveda and the Atharvaveda. For yoga students the most well-known is probably the Rigveda.

Epic Mahabharata

The Epic Mahabharata is a poem with 100 000 stanzas, includes the Bhagavad Gita and is much longer than the "Iliad" and the "Odyssey" together. However, over the years a lot of the original texts have not survived and today there are several modernised versions.

The Mahabharata includes texts covering mythology, religion, philosophy, ethics and customs. The "Gita" has always been enormously popular to the Indian people but also to Mahatma Gandhi as well as famous writers like Hegel, Schopenhauer, Walt Whitman, Christopher Isherwood and Aldous Huxley. The Gita which was first translated into English in 1785 has about 18 chapters on Hindu philosophy and advocates self-control, detachment and equanimity in all things.

Epic Ramayana

The Epic Ramayana (Rama's Journey) is an ancient poem of folk wisdom with 24 000 stanzas. It has influenced millions of people in India and abroad. There have been many TV versions watched by millions of viewers. It is a morality tale exploring moral values and virtues like duty and justice and the inherit order in Nature.

Yoga Sutras of Patanjali

So who was Patanjali? Apparently there have been many famous wise men of India with the same name. A lot of the information on Patanjali is purely speculative and he was probably a compiler of relevant texts rather than an original author. None the less, he is now regarded as the father of yoga and there are countless commentaries on his sutras. According to some authorities there are four sections of about 200 aphorisms and others say 195 or 196. The four sections or chapters are named Ecstasy or Contemplation, The Path or Practise, The Powers or Accomplishments and Liberation or Absoluteness.

For the serious student of yoga this book is an obvious first choice. It is easy to follow and has the fascinating advice right in the beginning that if you understand the second sutra then you already know what the rest of the book is all about and that the entire science of Yoga is based on this lesson.

The second sutra says: "The restraint of the wandering thoughts in the mind is Yoga."

The rest of the book provides instruction and advice on how to overcome difficulties, how to meditate, how to pursue Samadhi, how to quieten the mind etc.

One thing stands out that confirms the way Indian philosophy differs from western thinking. That is that the world is one's own projection and that there is little point in trying to change the outside world. This is impossible to take absolutely seriously for a westerner but surely contains some good advice on not getting too stressed about everything.

CHAPTER NINE

WISDOM WORDS

Some One-Liners can be seen as metaphors for yoga guidance. It is not difficult to find references with similar advice in yoga literature. Each and every one can be employed in concentrating the mind. Anyway, I found it fascinating to associate these wisdom words with the positive and life confirming practise of yoga.

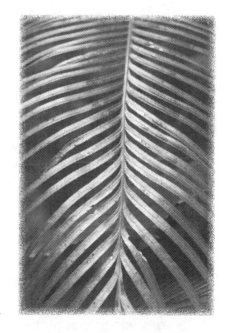

I like to try and remember that the brain has billions of cells and that each cell has hundreds of thousands of connections. Perhaps we can eliminate chaos of the mind and remove fear, insecurity, anger etc.

thereby making available larger mental resources. Strengthening both the mind and body with yoga practise will certainly cultivate a healthy life-style and may even slow down the aging process.

- Life stops when you stop dreaming
- Hope ends when you stop believing
- Nothing is worth it if you aren't happy
- You must love who you are, no one else will
- Walk away from unhappiness
- Life isn't about pleasing everybody
- Live now, most people just exist
- Respect yourself enough to walk away
- Don't let others destroy your confidence
- When you get to the end of your rope, tie a knot and hang on
- Life is a beautiful struggle
- A goal without a plan is just a wish
- Don't be pushed by your problems - be led by your dreams
- I want happiness. Remove the I (ego), want (desire) and happiness is left
- The world suffers, not because of evil people but because of silent good people
- Be authentic, genuine, real, yourself
- There are two mistakes on the truth road – not starting and not going all the way
- Never be bullied into silence. Neither allow yourself to be made a victim
- Celebrate your qualities
- Be you, don't apologize
- Find your passion

- Before yoga, something was always better than nothing. Now nothing is enough
- Associate with positive people
- Good friends are hard to find, harder to leave and impossible to forget
- People are lonely because they build walls instead of bridges
- Thoughts lead to words, actions, habits, character and then destiny

I have always felt that Wisdom cannot be taught or handed on to future generations. It has to be learnt over and over again. Otherwise there would have been only one war, one corrupt leader, one dictator, one psychopathic business executive, one river of refugees etc. It seems impossible for men and women to learn from the past.

Indian philosophy seems to have accepted the rather week standpoint that one can only change oneself and not society. Amnesty, Greenpeace, The Red Cross and Doctors Without Borders etc have all come from the Western world and they at least try and make a difference. It's difficult to see how such organisations could have come from India. However, world-wide yoga practise and meditation are deeply rooted in Indian philosophy and may provide a breakthrough and opportunity to stop the criminal madness of human beings. Each and every one of us can leave the yoga studio determined to bring Shanti into a universal oneness.

I tried to summarize Wisdom in my yoga poem I called **Your Yoga Journey.**

You have started a long journey,
          a yoga adventure.
Looking for awareness,
          looking for tranquillity.

You will start down wrong paths,
          through the maze of trying.
Yoga is your journey to new experiences.
          and new knowledge.

Your asanas will be messages,
          that will open doors.
To understanding,
          about yoga.

Sitting, standing, bending,
          movement and stillness.
Twisting, balancing, inverting,
          returning to unity.

The journey is everything,
          there is no arrival.
You will now have learnt,
          about wisdom.

That wisdom cannot be taught,
          that wisdom cannot be passed on.
That wisdom can only be drunk,
          from the Springs of Yoga.

CHAPTER TEN

Consciousness

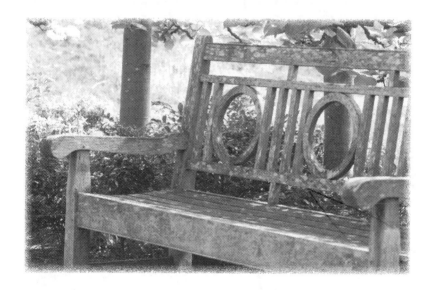

Beyond right and wrong, there is a garden. I will meet you there. (Rumi)

I feel it is hardly worthwhile in trying to exactly define the nature or concept of consciousness. Perhaps it is far better to admit that true consciousness is still undefinable but that it has been experienced by most people. The term consciousness is plagued by confused ideas and philosophies and self-awareness is just one of the very many goals. None the less, it can be helpful for a yogi student to compare the secular standpoint with the spiritual as found in the Indian philosophies. The yoga scholar is encouraged to strive and live the experience rather than get involved in endless debates on what is happening in the brain.

Secular Explanations

There are many different descriptions of consciousness, all trying to express and understand what is meant by the concept; medical experts, philosophers, scientists etc. have all tried to capture the feeling of heightened awareness or self-awareness or oneness. It is a matter of fact that many people experience something akin to these feelings when coming into a state of "flow" when everything is happening at the right time, in the right place and in perfect order. An athlete, a ballet dancer or an author can all experience a oneness which is very satisfying and which results in a perfect performance not otherwise obtainable. Going with the flow is an experience which one wants to continue for as long as possible. Perhaps this is the same as consciousness experienced during meditation.

In the beginning of my yoga practise I thought that I knew what consciousness was all about; a profound sense of relief and satisfaction after intensive yoga practise. These feelings persisted for several hours before being replaced by stress and the usual hustle and bustle of normal everyday life. However, I needed a more detailed clarification of what is happening when experiencing oneness.

Spiritual Explanation

The word spiritual seems to be the only term we can use to explain the experience of Samadhi in yoga. This is unfortunate due to the unfortunate use of the word by many so-called spiritual leaders. We can restrict it to encompass the experience of perfect harmony in yoga meditation. There are in fact many different states of Samadhi in Indian philosophy.

Ancient wise men from India have for generations been practising yoga as a means of becoming one with the object of meditation. They practised the famous forms called Raja yoga, Hatha yoga, Jnana yoga, Bhakti yoga, Karma yoga and Mantra yoga. There are many other modern yoga exercises developed and practised all over the world.

The sole purpose or goal of these yoga forms is to reach out beyond the everyday experience of just living and to try and attain self-realisation or what is known as Samadhi. There are countless descriptions and explanations of Samadhi but for my part glorious nothingness is good enough. I am not attracted to mystical or magical teachings. They all seem to end up with bitter disappointment.

Life itself does not appear meaningful and most of us would say that it is experienced as pure chaos. This attitude was encouraged by the wise yoga philosophers because it prompted a person to search for an individual solution to everyday problems without having to rely on the promise of another life after death. Life was created, experienced and extinguished over and over again in unending cycles. Surely, this is a very intelligent way of defining the experience of living.

The meaning and purpose of life first becomes apparent when we express something positive by our actions or thoughts. Yoga and meditation provide excellent techniques when searching for meaningfulness. The same might be said for religion but centuries of religious practise have failed to arrive at a universal ethic supporting a positive life view for both men and women. Many religions have included a superstitious belief in absurd teachings and the shameful interest in human blood rites or taboos which are still practised all over the world. There are still temples and churches which forbid the entrance of menstruating women.

Personally, I am attracted to yoga science as a superior way of replacing chaos in my life experience. So, it seems to me that yoga is a real alternative for reaching out to a more sensible way of living a full and true life. I like being fully responsible for my own searching and experimenting and not having to follow or obey some higher authority.

One thing has become very clear to me and that is the simple fact that intense spirituality can be experienced without the belief in any particular religion. Furthermore, that meditation can dive much deeper into the study of oneness or "Nothingness" than the doctrines of religion can offer.

It becomes apparent after a long lifetime that there are no absolute answers to questions about spirituality and that it is probably wiser to enjoy rather than expect otherwise. I suppose and hope that the majority of people would like to see the union of spiritualty with reason and ethics. In the meantime we yoga enthusiasts can enjoy the following experiences.

- A state of harmony
- A state of oneness
- A state of selflessness
- A state of nothingness
- A state of no passing thoughts
- Samadhi

We do not necessarily need to practise yoga to experience Samadhi and we do not need religion to explain that it is all a mystery. However, yoga asanas, meditation and pranayama all seem to heighten the experience. There is an element of pleasure in the search for consciousness. So all we have to do is to enjoy the adventure.

REFERENCE LITERATURE

The following is a short list with some of my favourite sources of knowledge on India and yoga. The 500-page "The Yoga Tradition by George Feuerstein" is highly recommended. This can be the beginning of a personal inward voyage.

The Yoga Tradition by George Feuerstein

Yoga Mind, Body & Spirit by Donna Farhi

The Yoga Sutras of Patanjali
(Commentary by Sri Swami Satchidananda)

Bhagavad Gita
(Commentary by Ram Dass in Living the Bhagavad Gita)

The Bhagavad Gita According to Gandhi by Mahatma Gandhi

Hatha Yoga Pradipika by Svatmarama
(Commentary by Hans Ulrich Rieker and foreword by BKS Iyengar)

Indian Thought and its Development by Albert Schweitzer

The Polair Illustrated Yoga Dictionary